I AM
A Journal for Internal Growth

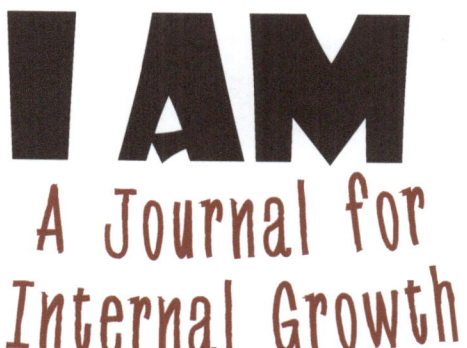

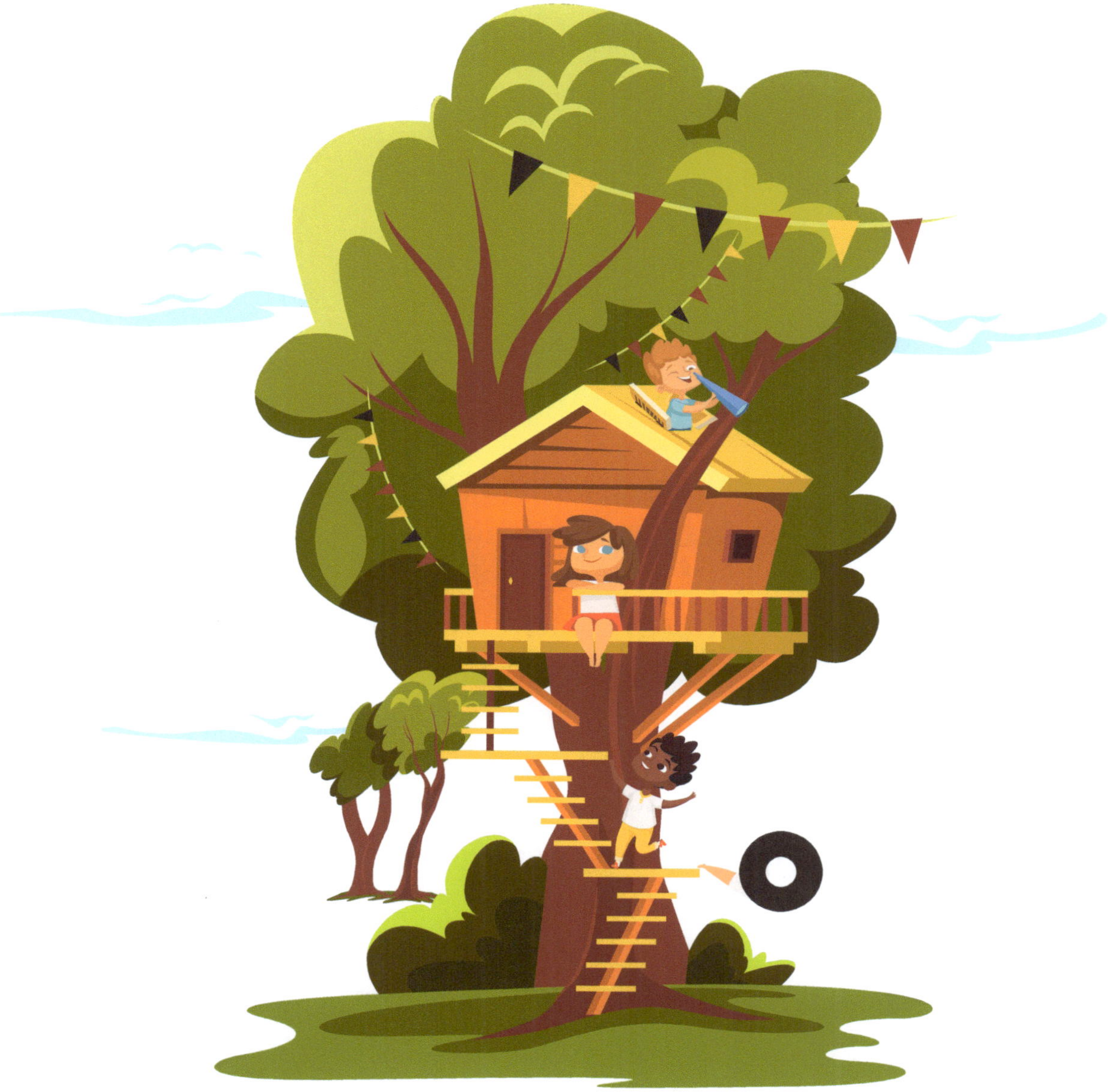

By Tracy Blom

I AM: A Journal for Internal Growth | 2022 All Rights Reserved
Author: Tracy Blom
No Part Of This Publication May Be Reproduced, Distributed, Or Transmitted In Any Form Or By Any Means, Including Photocopying, Recording, Or Other Electronic Or Mechanical Methods, Without The Prior Written Permission Of The Publisher, Except In The Case Of Brief Quotations Embodies In Critical Reviews And Certain Other Noncommercial Uses Permitted By Copyright Law

For permission requests, contact the author via her website:
www.theblomdotcom.com
Printed in the United States of America

This Journal Belongs To

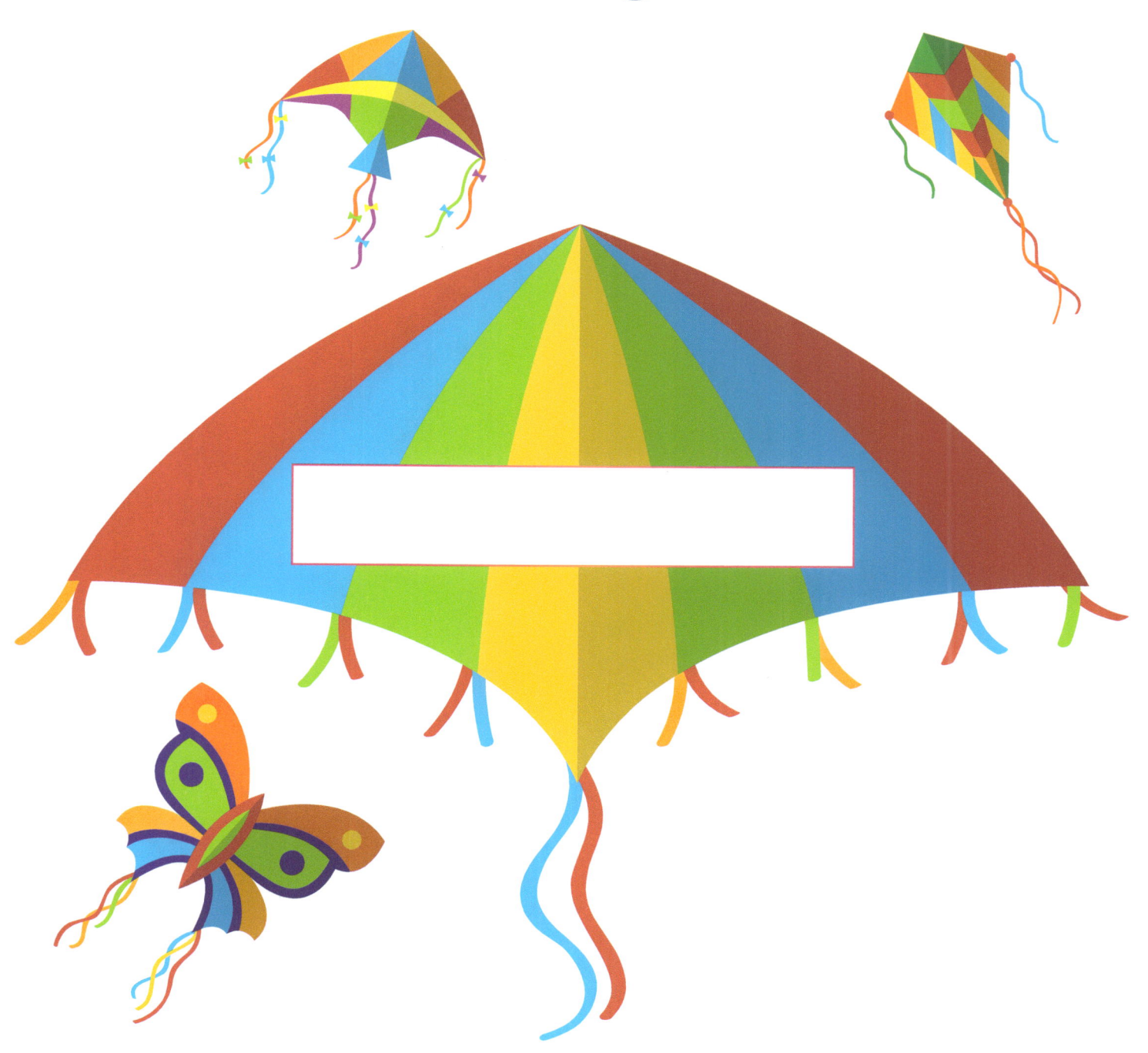

A Sense of Self

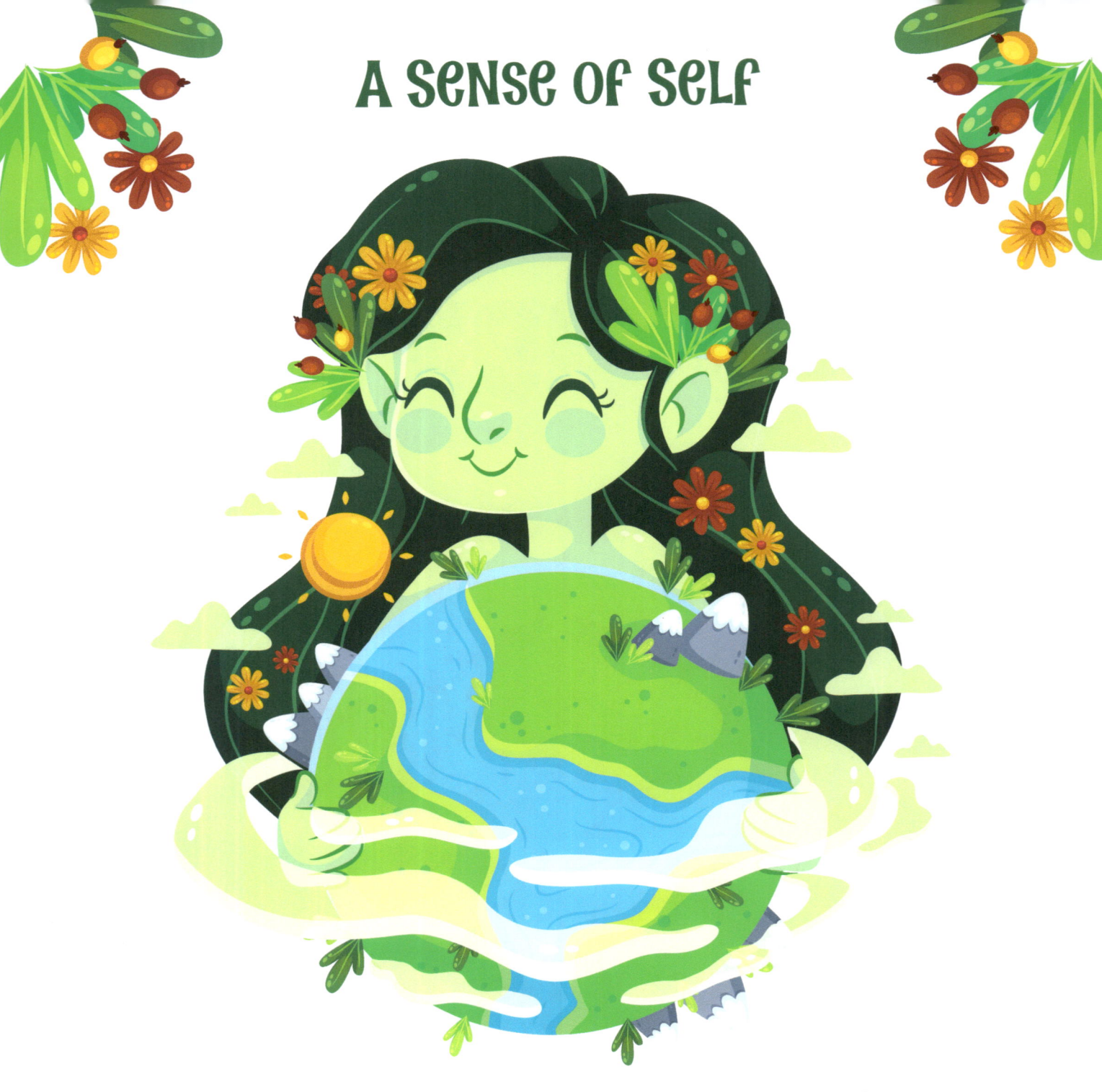

There are billions of people in the world, and everyone makes a difference... including YOU!
This journal is designed to be an outlet--- a place where you can explore your feelings and emotions openly and freely.

Let's start by talking about who you are.

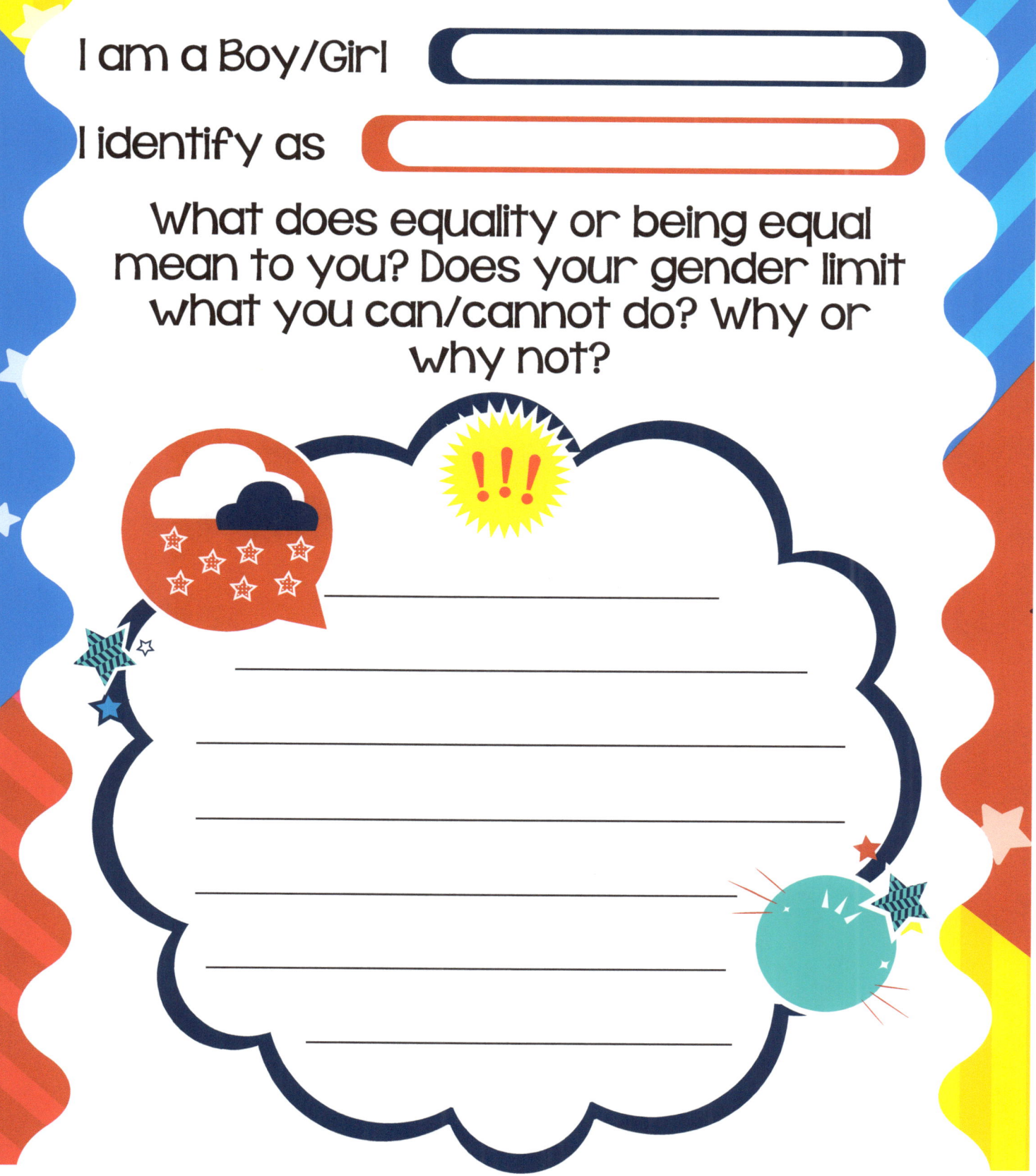

LET'S START BY TALKING ABOUT WHO YOU ARE.

I am a Boy/Girl

I identify as

What does equality or being equal mean to you? Does your gender limit what you can/cannot do? Why or why not?

SELF ACCEPTANCE

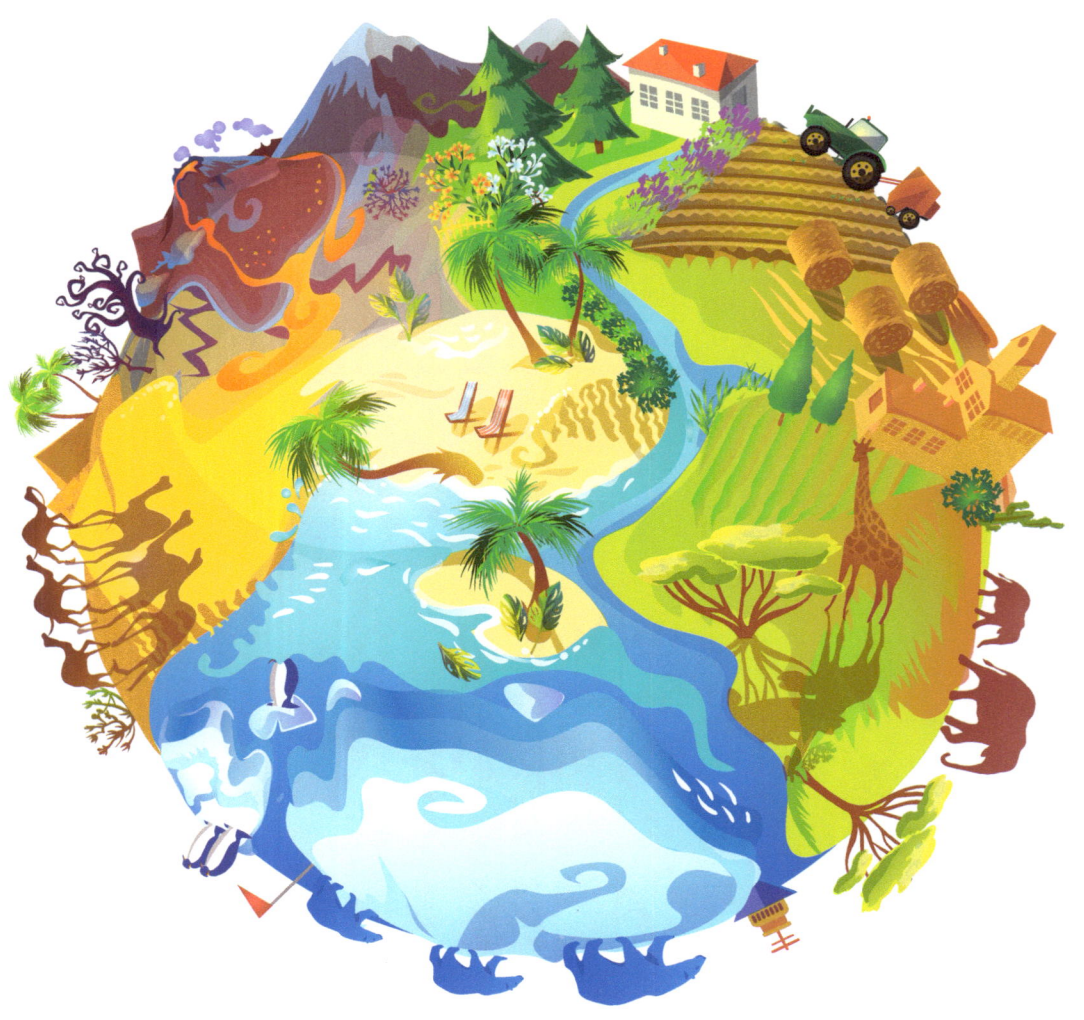

The world is round, filled with all races

With different cultures and lots of great

places!

I AM diverse

I AM unique

Love is the language that I speak!

Affirmation:
"I AM self-acceptance. I AM perfectly me."

When you look in the mirror, what do you see?
(beauty, flaws, perfection, strength)

_____
_____
_____
_____

How do you feel when you look at yourself?
(self-love, happiness, sadness)

_____
_____
_____

Why do you feel this way?

_____
_____
_____
_____

What qualities do you have that
make you unique?

_____
_____
_____

HERITAGE

Our differences are what make us unique! From the clothes that we wear to the language we speak.

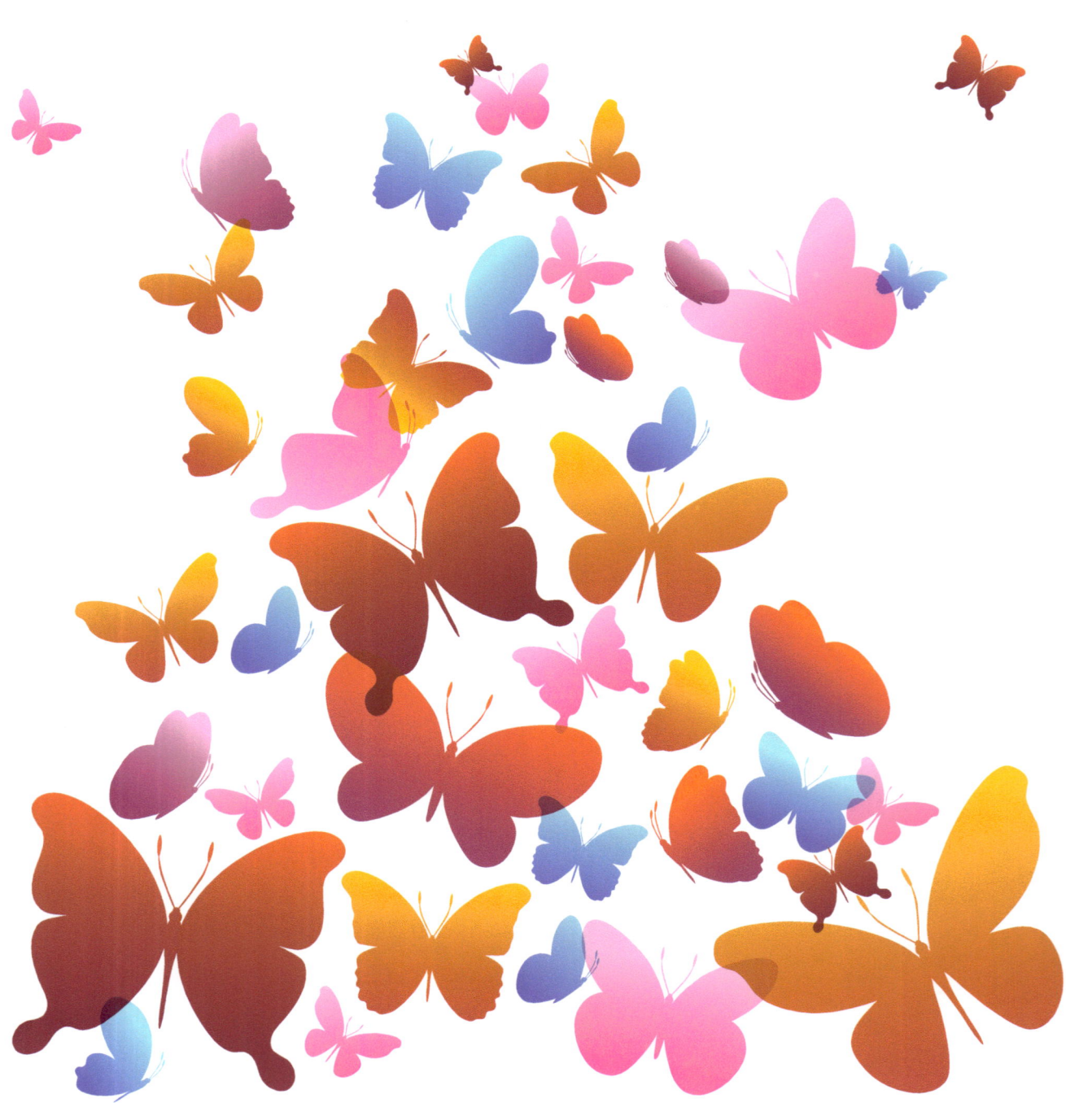

What family traditions do you have?
_____
_____
_____

Do you, or anyone in your family speak another language?
_____
_____
_____

I am friends with people who look like me or don't look like me?
_____
_____
_____

Why or why not?
_____
_____
_____

What qualities do you look for in a friend? (nice, caring, funny)
_____
_____
_____

What are the three most important things that people should know about you?
_____
_____
_____

KINDNESS MATTERS

Every good deed, both big and small,

Creates *change* in the world and goodness for ALL!
What have YOU done, or what could YOU do,

To make the world BETTER for me and for you?

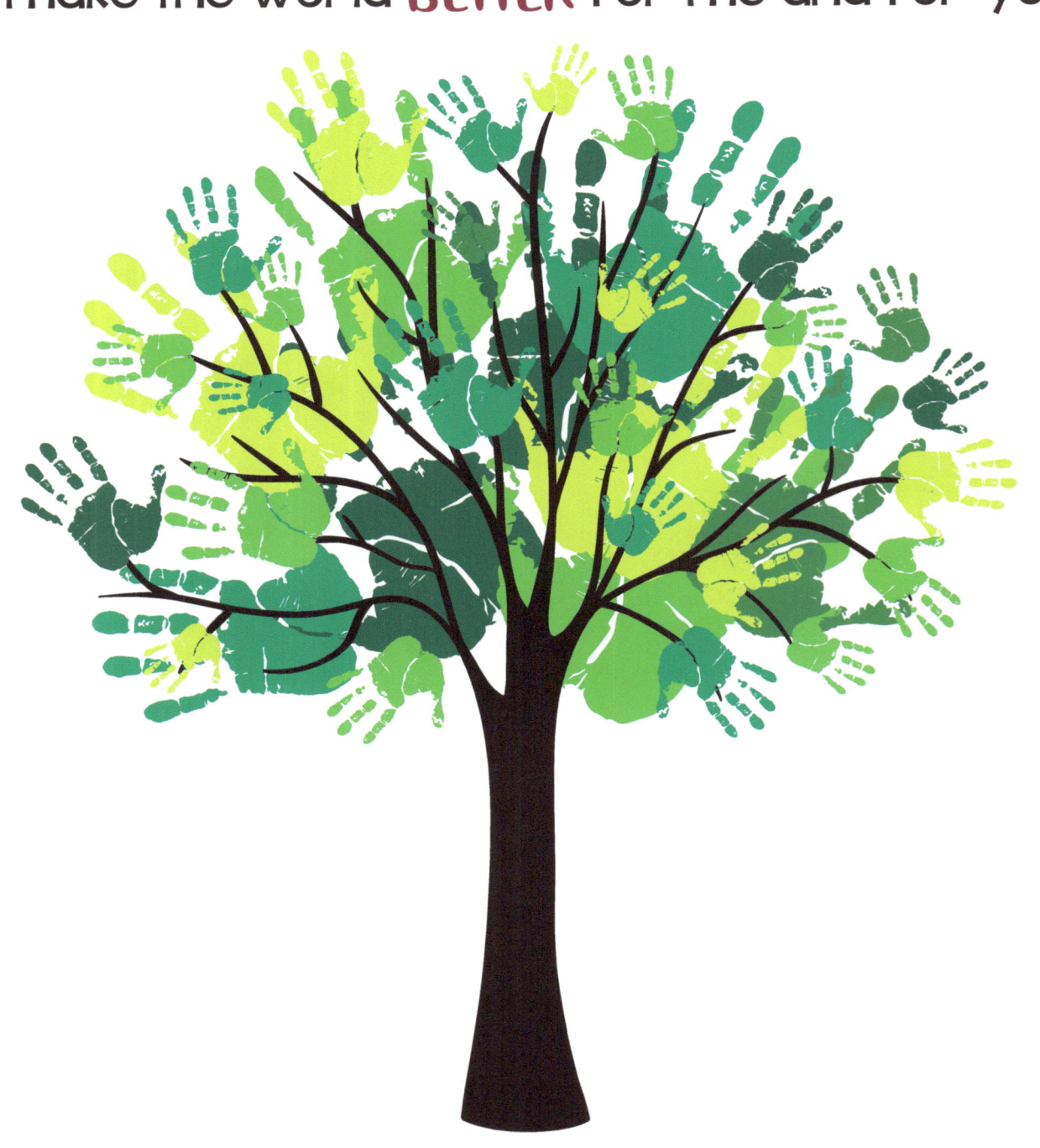

Have you ever made someone's day better? How?

Do you think that good deeds matter? Why?

If you could change one thing in the world, what would it be?

Do you believe that you can create change? Can you do this alone, or as a group? Or both?

I wonder how the spider, so *tiny* and small, can make a web so **STRONG** and so tall?
One of the nature's small creatures, holds silk inside, and helps to clothe people far and wide,
Have you underestimated yourself?
Your **ABILITIES** are not measured by size, age or wealth

Do you believe in yourself?

___

Name a goal you would like to achieve in the next month

- ___
- ___
- ___

Are there reasons why you feel you can't achieve your goal?

___

Let's try something fun! Close your eyes, and envision achieving your goal. Do this every day for just a few moments, and see if this helps!

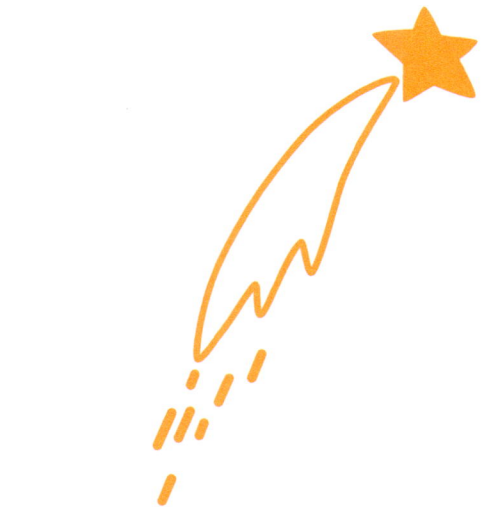
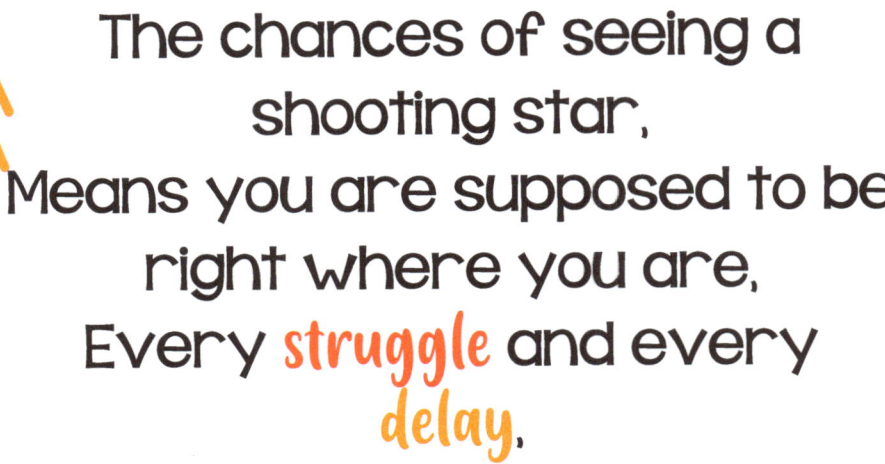

The chances of seeing a shooting star,
Means you are supposed to be right where you are,
Every **struggle** and every **delay**,
Is a **LESSON** that you can learn today
Can you look at your challenges from a different view?
As a way to learn something **new**?

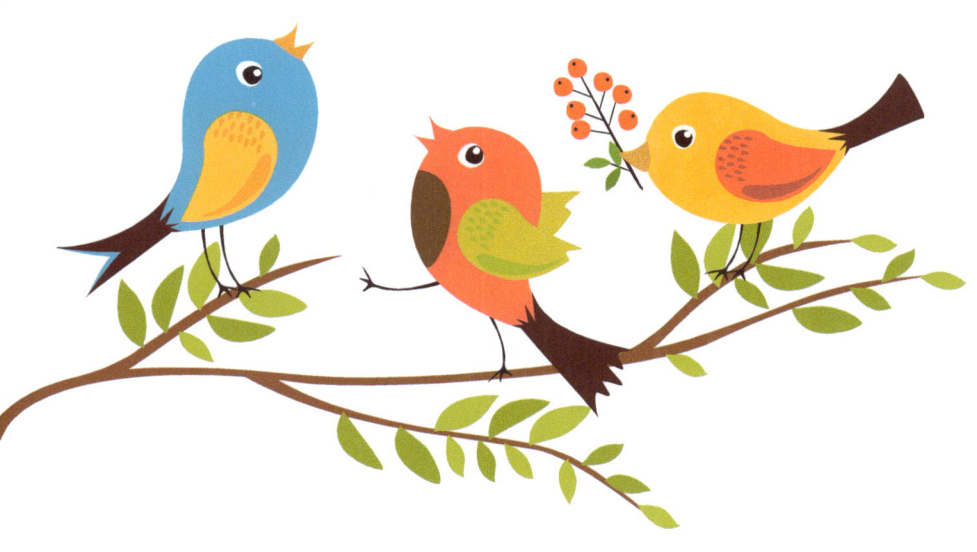

Describe a situation that turned out to be good.
Example: My bike got a flat tire and I walked to school, and that is how I met my best friend.

_____
_____
_____
_____

Do you think there is a lesson in your story above?

_____
_____
_____
_____

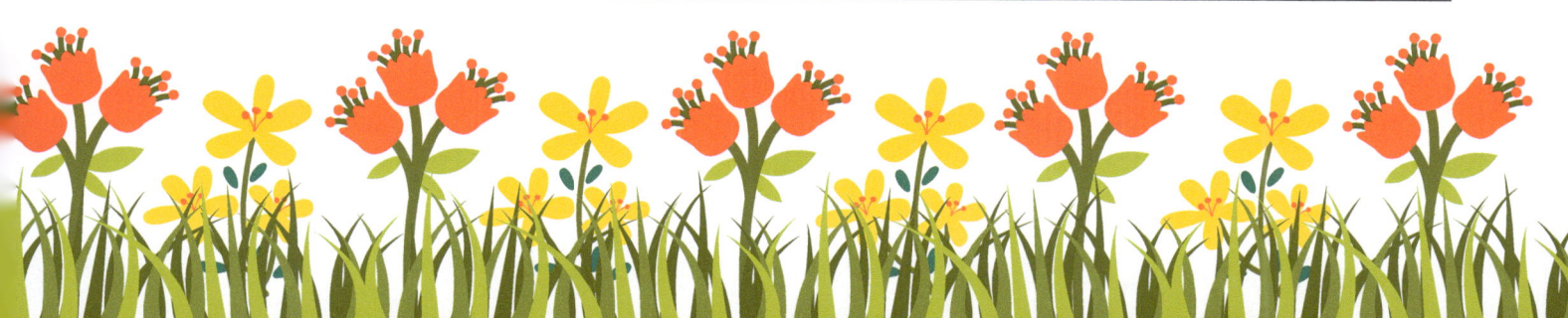

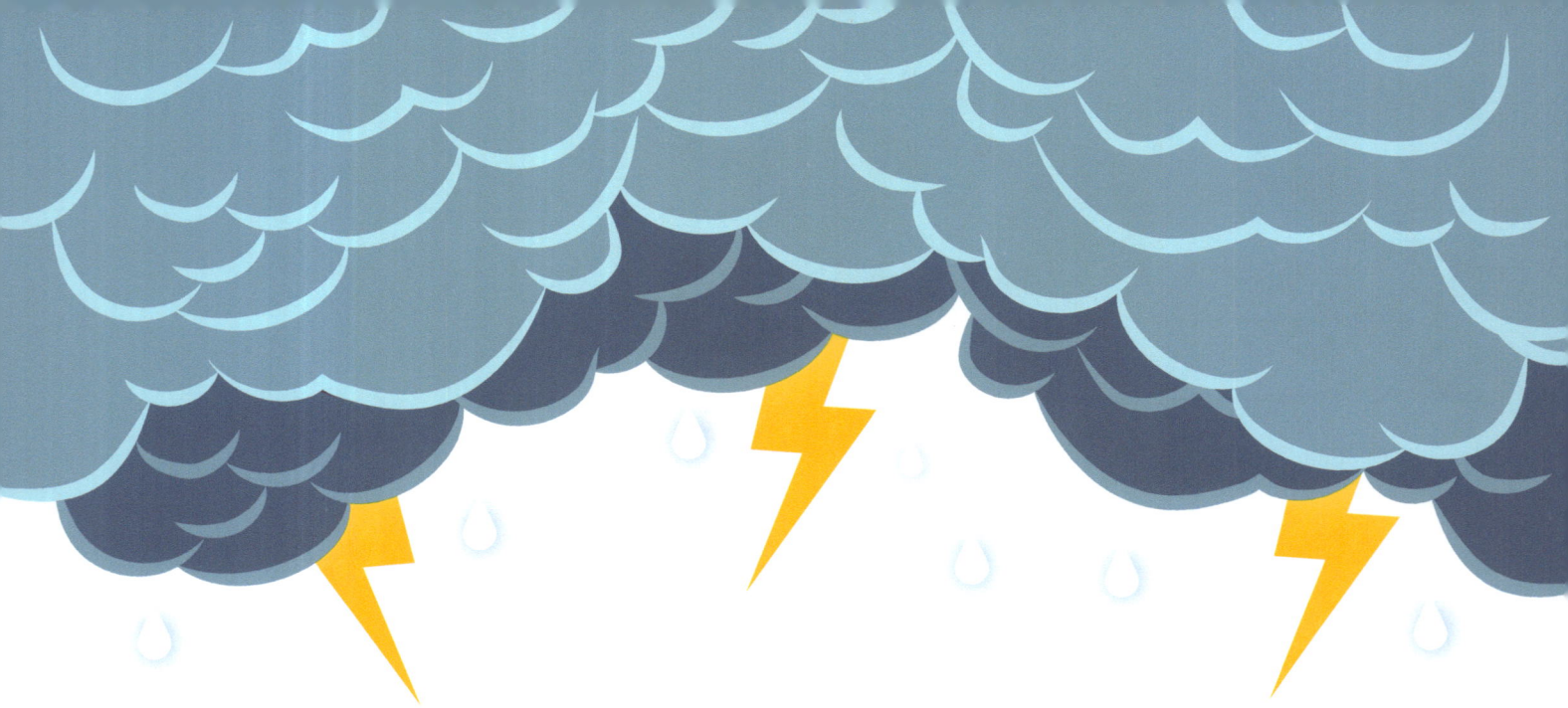

There may be a STORM outside,
But the safest place to run and hide,
Is a CALM, clear place within your MIND
Is this a place that you can find?

When you face trouble, stress, sadness or anger, what do you do? Why?

_____
_____

How do you find peace during a hard time? (talk to someone you love, listen to music,

_____
_____

Can you create peace for yourself, and for others?

_____
_____

Let's try something fun! Next time you are upset, move to a quiet place and take five

Exercise One: Find a person at school that you've never talked to before, and try to get to know them. Below, write what you learned about them?

_____
_____
_____
_____

Exercise Two: How can you make the planet a better place? Describe your activity below, and how you felt when you did it. Example: plant a tree or flower, pick up trash, recycle!

_____
_____
_____
_____

Exercise Three: Take five minutes to sit in silence without your phone, or any other device. How does silence make you feel? (if your mind starts racing, try taking a few deep breaths and focus on your breathing instead.)

_____
_____
_____
_____
_____

Exercise Four: Come up with a way to bring joy to someone else, unexpectedly, without them asking for it. What did you do? How did this make you feel when you did it?

_____
_____
_____
_____
_____

Is there a talent that you wish you had? What are some things you could do to practice?

_____
_____
_____
_____
_____
_____
_____
_____
_____
_____
_____
_____
_____
_____
_____

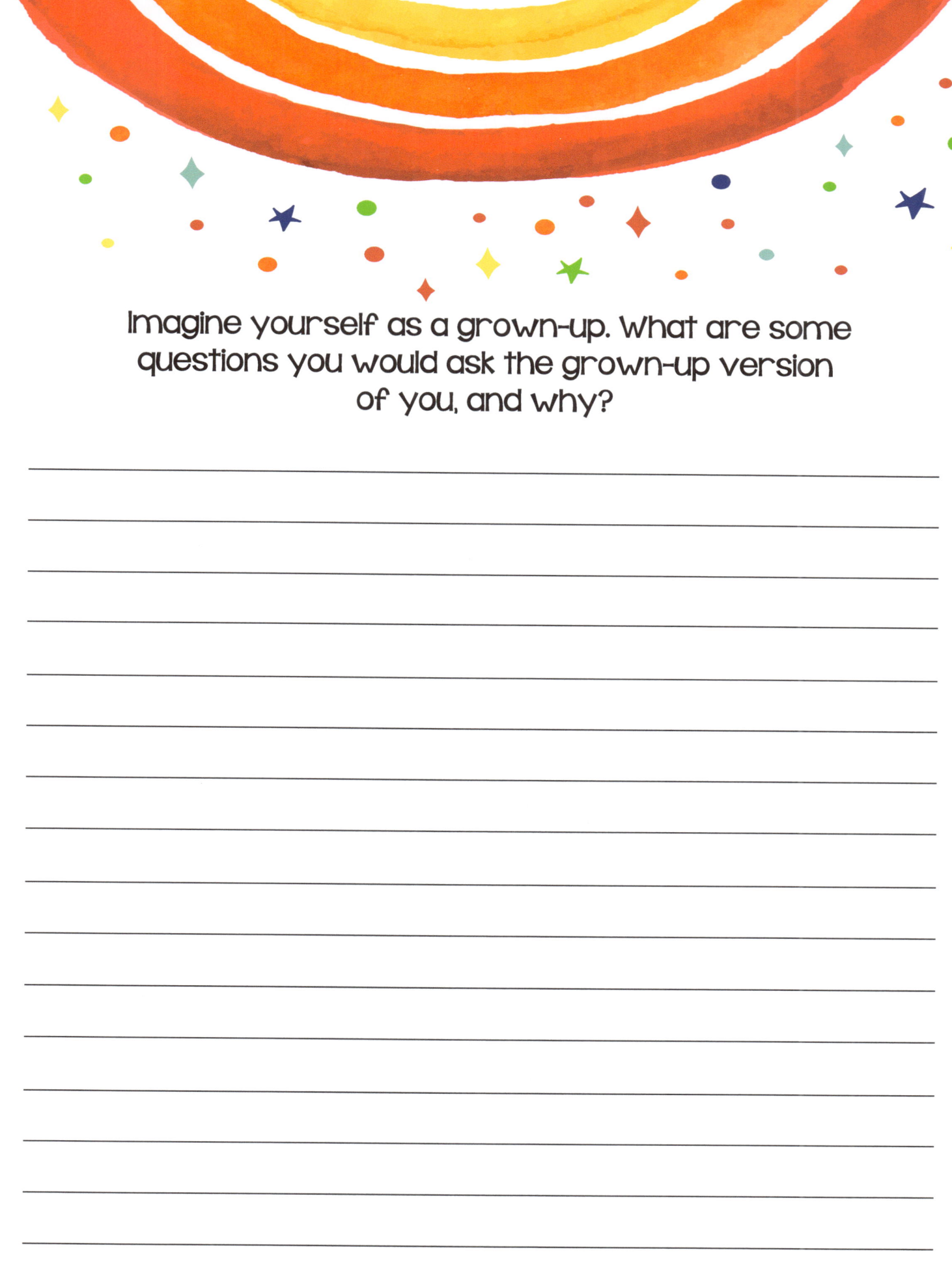

Imagine yourself as a grown-up. What are some questions you would ask the grown-up version of you, and why?

_____
_____
_____
_____
_____
_____
_____
_____
_____
_____
_____
_____

In this exercise I invite you to learn about where you live. What trees grow in your town, what birds and animals exist there, and what did the land look like a hundred years ago?

___
___
___
___
___
___
___
___
___
___
___
___
___
___
___
___
___
___
___
___
___

If there was one place in the world that you could visit, where would you go? Why?

_____
_____
_____
_____
_____
_____
_____
_____
_____
_____
_____
_____
_____
_____
_____
_____